SEX

A Modern Sex Guide to Pleasuring your Partner

ALICIA BELLEROSE

Table of Contents

INTRODUCTION

Congratulations on downloading *Sex: A Modern Guide to Pleasuring your Partner* and thank you for doing so.

The following chapters will discuss how to please your partner. It will provide tips and tricks to bringing some serious steam to the bedroom. The first half of the book will discuss ways to pleasure a man while the second will provide ways to pleasure a woman. A little later on, there are going to be some additional chapters on sex that is not really talked about on a regular basis. We will provide you with some taboo type ideas to bring some excitement to you and your partner.

Before we get down to the nitty gritty of this book about sex, prepare yourself to read words that most are uncomfortable saying out loud. Once you are really comfortable with your partner, you could discover that they might like to hear those words whispered in their ear. Try not to blush and read on. It is going to be great!

There are plenty of books on this subject on the market, thanks again for choosing this one! Every effort was made to ensure it is full of as much useful information as possible, please enjoy!

PLEASURE TRIGGERS FOR HIM

There may have been those who elude to the fact men are *easy* to please. That may be the case for some men, but certainly not true for all. That being said, there are areas on a man's body that are known as *feel-good* zones. Sex experts have discovered that men typically have nine of these areas that you should know about if you want to really give him sexual gratification. These zones might even be unknown to your partner. They are literal hot spots that are jam-packed with ultra-sensitive nerve endings, all of which will really get him going once they have been stimulated. The nine zones are listed below. There will also be specific ideas on where to lick, stroke and squeeze to really push your man into orgasmic bliss.

The first of these erogenous zones might come as a surprise. It is the **lower lip**. It does not include the entire lip, however. There is a slope that can be found in between the outside of his lower lip and chin that is incredibly sensitive. That little curve is full of super sensitive nerve receptors. While making out with your man, suck the lower lip and pull it into your mouth. Then, utilize the tip of your tongue by stroking it up and down that little curve just below his lip. That move arouses that entire zone in such a sexually provoking manner that it will really get him excited. By keeping that lower lip of his in your mouth, the sensation is amplified. This motion will make him feel as though little electrical currents surge straight from his mouth down to his shaft.

The second zone is the **front of the neck**. When it comes to this area, we tend to lick or suck on the side of the neck near the ears. Another area we tend to focus on is the collarbone. Those might work just fine, but it is not an area full of those sensitive nerves. The major point of stimulation is the spot just beneath the Adam's apple. Medical professionals refer to it as the thyroid. It is a gland shaped like a butterfly that is a little more than halfway down the front of the neck. It is linked, quite closely, to the sex organs, so says Chinese medicine practitioners. To activate this zone, you will want to have him lie down on his back. It is best to have a pillow behind his head so that his neck is arched forward ever so slightly and that Adam's apple is exposed. Tease him just a little by brushing your lips against the lowest part of his throat. (known as the hollow) After that, use the flat part of your tongue and slide it upward until you reach the Adam's apple. Because the thyroid is directly beneath it, dip back down slightly. Massage the whole area using circular, wide motions with the tongue. Those circles ensure the entire thyroid is covered, which gives him the maximum amount of pleasure. By the time you are done with him, he will be incredibly hot and bothered.

The third zone might sound like it is more geared toward a woman. Surprisingly enough, a man's **nipples** could be even more sensitive than those of a woman. This is likely due to the fact men are not used to having their nipples be the center of sexual attention. Most men's nipples are like uncharted territory in that they are erogenous zones that have yet to be experimented with. Touching them will send pleasurable shock waves throughout his entire body. The best trick with the nipples is known as the *ice cream swirl.* While he lays on his back, you will lick slow circles around the outside of his nipple. Start at the areola and make slow circles moving inward until you reach the nipple. This is a very tantalizing move with the tongue. Once you reach the nipple, give it a little flick with the tip of your tongue and then nip it ever so gently. Building up pleasure in that manner is something that men truly love. If you'd like to up the ante a little, suck on an ice cube for a while before you start. The coldness of your tongue supercharges the nerve endings of the nipple.

Another zone that might come as a surprise is the dip just underneath his **ankle.** This point is found about halfway between the ankle bone and heel. The pressure point is about the size of your fingertip and it has some serious erogenous potential. Amazingly enough, it is another area directly linked to your man's sex organ. By pressing into it, energy is released and produces pleasurable feelings as a result. The best way to literally get your man to blow a gasket is to ride your man in reverse (this move is called the reverse cowgirl). When you feel him near climax, reach down and grab his ankles. Put a little bit of pulsating pressure on the ankle in time with his thrusts.

The next zone we are going to cover is the **perineum.** Many men tend to be a little shy when it comes to talking about this area, or guiding you to it. It is the patch of skin just behind his sac. Beneath that is the prostate gland which is an organ with quite a bit of orgasmic power. Rubbing that gently will bring him to the brink of climax rather quickly. Just before he prepares to enter you, take his sac into your hands and rub them lightly. While your hand is down there, press the knuckles gently against the perineum. While you two are getting down and dirty, keep rubbing and kneading. Just as he is about to climax, press your knuckles a little deeper. That move will lengthen and intensify his orgasm.

It may seem that the **shaft** does not need mentioning. However, there is one move in particular that will really set your man on fire. For this particular move, have your man lay down comfortably on his back. Sit between his legs (they should be outstretched) and face him. Take your thumb and index finger and make two tight rings around his shaft. One will be at the top while the other is in the middle. Slide your *rings* in opposing directions moving from the base to the head moving both hands simultaneously. There will be tantalizing friction, especially if things start off particularly slow and teasingly. Speed up only to slow down again to add to the sexual tension. Lubricant isn't required, but it will make this action much more pleasurable for him, so give it a try. Either way, he is going to love it.

Mentioning the shaft brings us to the next part of the penis and that is the **head.** There are more receptors for pleasure at the head than in any other part of the penis. It can be difficult to apply the right amount of pressure. The kind that brings him sexual bliss, not the kind that makes him want to keep your mouth permanently away from his package. There is a specific maneuver you can use called *the lipstick trick.* To accomplish this, you will have your man lie on his back, his stiff member pointing upward. Take hold of the base with your fingers to hold him steady. Make sure you aren't using a fist, just the fingers. Keep your lips closed yet relaxed as you brush them against the head. Rub it over your wet mouth in a motion mimicking the application of lipstick. This sensation can be heightened by opening your lips slightly and rubbing the head in between them. On occasion, take the entire head into your mouth, then return to just rubbing the head against your lips. He will love being able to watch as you tease him with your luscious lips.

You know the crease on the **testicles** that seems to act as a partition for the boys? That is known as the seam and is one of the erogenous zones we are going to cover in this book. Apparently, it has a lot more pleasure sensors than we originally thought. In order to get to those super sensitive places, you will need to once again take the initiative. This area is sensitive though, so tread lightly. Take his sac in one hand, then gently press your index finger and middle finger of the other hand into the top part of the crease. This will be closest to where the sac meets the base of the penis. Trace a line down with your fingers until you get to the bottom of the scrotum. While still massaging with one hand, slide your fingers back up to the top once more. Those movements are sure to get him really aroused.

The last zone we are going to talk about in this chapter is the **frenulum.** Known as the *F spot*, it is the area of flesh that sits just under the crown of the penis and is where the shaft meets the head. It does not get much for attention, perhaps because it is not very noticeable, especially when the penis is fully erect. In order to excite him with this *F spot,* you will take the base of his penis in one hand and lick slow circles around the crown. Every time you circle back around to that frenulum, flick your tongue quickly over it a couple of times, then go back to licking circles around the crown. All the while, you will continue to work your hand up and down the shaft. This maneuver is sure to give him a mind-blowing orgasm.

FOREPLAY FOR HIM

Sometimes, life gets in the way and some of us still want to please our man, but there just is not enough time in the day. On occasion, it is easier just to let your man have a quickie and that is okay every once in a while. Doing something like that all the time will make the bedroom boring for the both of you. In the long run, that can lead to issues in the relationship. This book is meant to focus on more pleasurable things, however. Without further ado, we are going to talk about foreplay.

Foreplay can build sexual tension and ultimately heighten the pleasure felt during sex. It can be a fun way to get both your engines revved. There are lots of different forms of foreplay that may not actually involve touching your man. For instance, something as simple as leaving the lights on is a form of foreplay. Men tend to be very visual creatures and they are often turned on by what they see. Undress slowly while he watches. Perhaps wear some naughty lingerie underneath for an added surprise.

Believe it or not, dressing sexy is also foreplay. If the two of you have a party to go to, or just plan on going out to a bar for drinks, dress sexy! That alone is going to get him thinking about peeling those clothes off when the two of you get back home. Another good tip is to make sure the downtown is nice and neat. Shaving or waxing is an easy way to keep things tidy and men love to see a well maintained kitty on a woman. Take this a step further and tell him that you have shaved before the two of you leave the house. It will having him thinking about that all night as well. Both those are going to build an incredible sexual tension between the two of you.

Another form of foreplay is to talk dirty. In today's world, there are so many ways in which we can communicate, it makes it easy for us to spice it up. Dirty talk builds sexual tension long before the two of you make it into the bedroom. You can send text messages while he's at work so that he is thinking about all the things you are going to do to him when he gets home. You can also press your body against his and whisper sweet, dirty somethings into his ear. If you find yourself in need of ideas to get you started, look no further. Below are a few phrases that will help get your creative (and other) juices to flow.

We will start out with a few text message examples and then we will give you some ideas of what to say in the bedroom and even during sex.

Text Messages:

1. I woke up so wet this morning.

2. I am not wearing any panties.

3. I love the way your dick tastes.

4. I am in bed…naked and waiting for you.

5. I can't wait for you to be inside me tonight.

The thing with text messages is you do want to keep them short and sweet, definitely to the point. Those examples listed above are teasers. They are going to get your man thinking about sex with you later that evening. What is great about text messages is they build a lot of sexual tension without the two of you being anywhere near each other. Those are just a few ideas for you to get started. It really is a great way to tease your man from afar and get you excited in the process.

Dirty talk in the bedroom:

1. I'm so wet right now.

2. I need you inside me now!

3. I love the way your body feels on top of mine.

4. I want you to spank me. (Men like to pull hair too, use that as well).

5. Take me right here, right now, any way you want.

Those are some beginner comments to make while in the bedroom with your man. Obviously, you know your man best so you can gauge the level of dirty depending on what he likes and does not like. Have fun with this. It is really a great way to stimulate your man and heighten the pleasure the both of you feel during sex.

We are going to give you a few more tips on talking dirty face to face before we move on to more physical foreplay. They are really easy and will drive home the dirty talk messages.

1. Look him in the eyes when you are speaking. It is an intimate and sexy way to help convey your message. It shows that you are confident and serious about the things you are saying. If you are really shy, try practicing in front of a mirror a few times before you try these phrases out on your man.

2. Keep your breaths even and speak in a seductive tone. There is no need to go for an Oscar and overact when you are attempting to talk dirty, but a little softer tone with a kick of seduction in your voice is going to really turn your man on.

3. If you are nervous about saying these things face to face, you can also talk dirty to him while you rub his shoulders. Giving him a pre-game massage while whispering dirty messages in his ear is really exciting to a man.

Finally, remember that talking dirty can also be you telling him what you want him to do to you during sex. Something as simple as, *fuck me harder* can really encourage your man and get him going.

Now we are going to get into some foreplay tips using touch. Start out small. If the two of you are sitting on the couch watching television, start rubbing his scalp. This is actually a move that can be used before, during and after foreplay. It is not one of the erogenous zones we talked about in the previous chapter, but men do enjoy having their big head rubbed just as much as the little one. Start out lightly brushing your fingers across his scalp, then gradually apply a little more pressure. During sex, while he is on top, rub his scalp some more to really add to the pleasure.

Another great thing to do is to take charge by taking hold of his penis. Before the two of you even get naked, you can press your body up against him and rub him through his pants. After the two of you are naked, take the foreplay further by having him lie on his back and you rub your moist lips up and down his stiff member. Once he is good and hard, take his penis and hold it upright. Slide just the tip in and out several times. Both of these are a lot of fun and they work to get the both of you even more excited.

The next foreplay tip is that of kissing. It may not sound like much, but when done correctly, it really does the trick. Kissing your man with intensity and passion is a huge turn on and is ridiculously hot. Taking the initiative and kissing your man first is a giant step in the right direction. Men do not always like to be the initiator. By you giving him a hot, aggressive kiss it shows

19

you really are interested in having sex and not just doing so to keep him happy.

A few things you can do to increase the intensity of your kiss are to suck his bottom lip into your mouth. Give it a little tug while your eyes are locked on his. You can even nibble the bottom lip. Just make sure to keep it gentle. Nothing will ruin the mood quicker than a bleeding lip. While kissing, use that scalp massage technique we talked about previously. While rubbing his head, you can also direct his head whichever way you please. Tilting it slowly from one side to the other as you kiss him deeply puts you in control and is great for foreplay. Move from his lips to his jaw line, nibble on the ear lobe, kiss the collar bone and come back up to his lips. Your man has a lot of kissable places on his body. Take some time to get to know them with your lips. He will love it.

Using your hands and using them well is another awesome foreplay technique. There are several things you can do with your hands *before* you even get down to his package. With your palms flat against his chest, rub from his pecs all the way down to his abs. Run your finger just underneath his undies and tease the base of his shaft before moving your hands back up his body. You can also lightly scratch him. Using the same technique as above, rake your nails lightly over his chest and abs. When you go back up, drag them down over his shoulders and his arms. It does often tickle men, but it is a good tickle. Just make sure to apply the right amount of pressure. Too deep will leave painful scratch marks and too light will not give him the *right* kind of tickle.

The last subject we are going to tackle in the way of foreplay for your man is the blowjob. Men absolutely love watching you take them into your mouth and lick and suck their throbbing shaft. Begin by teasing him a little. Take his penis into your hand and stroke him gently. Kiss him anywhere and everywhere around the penis without actually taking it into your mouth. This is going to build up a lot of tension. Kiss his upper thigh, his abdomen, lick on the inside of the thigh right next to his sac. After you have teased him a bit, start to kiss his member from the tip to the bottom of the shaft. From there, incorporate a little tongue action. Lick up and down, give the tip a little flick with the tongue and then take just the tip into your mouth. Tease him like that a few moments before taking all of him (or as much as your mouth can handle) between your lips.

As you are sucking, massage his shaft with the flat part of your tongue. When you get back up to the tip, swirl your tongue around the head before going back down. All the while, massage his sac or you can also have one hand around the base of his shaft and massage that while you suck. Listen to the sounds he makes. You do not want to apply too much pressure with your mouth or your hands. You also want to avoid scraping with the teeth. A little bit is good, just be careful not to overdo it.

SPICING IT UP! SEXUAL POSITIONS FOR HIM

As stated in the previous chapter, life can often get busy and we find ourselves having sex quickly so that we can get back to doing what we need to live. Work, kids, family obligations...they all require our time and brain power which makes us tired at the end of the day. Even in the instance of a *quickie,* you can change sexual positions to make it more enjoyable for the both of you. The topics we are going to cover in this chapter are geared more toward longer lovemaking, but they can be used in a quick afternoon romp as well.

The first position we will talk about is you being on top. Previously, we discussed taking control during foreplay and this position can help you take control during sex. It makes you the driver and it is just where your man wants you to be. As the one on top, you get to set the pace and ride him as slow or as fast as you please. Bring his hands to your breasts and encourage him to caress them. An added tip here is to leave the lights on and let him see exactly what he is working with. As previously stated, men are highly visual beings. The ability to see you while you are in control is going to drive him absolutely wild.

Next, a position we touched on briefly during the erogenous zones chapter is that of the *reverse cowgirl.* This is still done with the woman on top, but facing away from her man. This gives your man the view of that ass he loves so much and the ability to see exactly what is going on while you ride him in reverse. You are still in control and while this position does not allow much in the way of eye contact, it does give him the opportunity to give a few smacks to the rear. Every once in a while, take a look over your shoulder and cast him a sexy glance. He will love it.

Doggie style is a position that lets your man be in complete control. He can set the pace, depth and rhythm that he enjoys most. This position allows him to go deeper, which is great for the both of you. That being said, sometimes it can be slightly uncomfortable for the woman. The key to great sex for the both of you is communication. Tell him what you like and do not like about this position. You can also raise or lower your hips to adjust how deep he can go. Adjusting the width of your knees on the bed is also helpful.

Another variation of doggie style is to lie down flat on your stomach. This is best done while your man is still inside you. This position presses your butt up against him and it lessens the depth of his strokes. Also, your clit rubs on the bed which adds to the pleasure you feel while he is having his way from behind.

Standing up is one of those positions that are done in the heat of the moment. It is one of those sexy, must have him now type of positions that makes him feel sexy and irresistible. It is a great variation to use for a spontaneous (or even planned) quickie. If the kids are not present, let him take you up against the kitchen counter or bent over the table. Up against a wall or the bedroom door are also perfect. If flexibility allows, have him drape one leg over his arm so he can drive upward and go a little deeper as well.

Spooning has more sexual value than just lying in bed, fully clothed and cuddling. It is a great way to start, though! Rub your but up against him and get him in the mood. Once the clothes are off, keep in this position. There are a few variations that are a lot of fun. You can stay in the traditional spooning position. You can also lift the top leg over his hips to allow for deeper penetration. With your leg up over his hips, it provides either or both of you access to your clit to further stimulate the both of you. In this position, either of you can be in charge. If you want to take control, put your hand on his hip and hold him still while you milk him slowly.

Another position that will drive your man crazy is called the sidewinder. This is kind of like spooning but you get to make eye contact and kiss. In this position, you will lie down on your sides so that you are facing each other. Lift your top leg and allow him to enter you. From there, wrap that top leg around his. An added bonus for him here is for you to keep your legs closer together, which makes it tighter for him and adds to his pleasure.

Eyes to the sky is great for men. In this position, you are going to start off by doing the reverse cowgirl. From there, lean back slowly (you want to make sure the transition is smooth. Moving too fast can cause him to fall out and if it is mid stroke, that might cause a bit of pain for the both of you) Keep leaning back until your back is flat on his chest and the both of you face the ceiling. This makes for more skin to skin contact and he will be able to touch anywhere on the front part of your body he pleases.

The waterfall is an incredibly intense move for your man. You will have him lie down on his back with his head and shoulders hanging down onto the floor. It can be uncomfortable for your man if he has to hold the position too long, so it is best to save this one for last. The rush of blood to his brain will make his climax much more intense. All the while, he gets to watch while you do the work.

The lotus is another great position geared toward pleasing your man. For this, the two of you will be sitting upright. You are going to straddle him and wrap your legs around his back. It is incredibly intimate and allows him to go deeper than he could in almost any other position. Either of you can be in control while in the lotus, but your man will love the feeling of you taking control and riding him at your pace. In this position, he will have a full view and access to your taut nipples and the two of you can engage in some passionate, mildly aggressive kissing as well.

If you really want to tease and please your man, go for the lap dance position. This is a fun one. You can start out wearing something sexy. Have your man sit in a chair. If you like, have some music playing in the background to add to the sexy factor. While he is sitting, give him a lap dance and peel off that sexy outfit you donned slowly. Once nude, you can ride him in reverse or facing him. While facing him, the two of you can make eye contact, kiss and you can rub your breasts up against him. In reverse, he can look down and watch as you take control. Either way, your man is going to be able to let his hands roam freely while getting pleasure from you.

The last position we are going to recommend for your man is called the pretzel. It might be one you have never heard of and if not, your man is going to absolutely love it. You will lay down on your side with your bottom leg outstretched and flat. Raise the top leg and wrap it around his waist. Your man is going to kneel, his legs will straddle your outstretched bottom leg. From there, he will enter you and can use his arm or hand to keep that top leg up in the air while he thrusts. This angle is going to give the both of you a fantastic view, which is a major turn on for your man. Neither of you are in complete control which means you are going to need to work together to find a pleasurable rhythm that will send the both of you over the edge.

To close up this chapter, we are going to touch on a few extra things that are going to really please your man. In addition to foreplay, there are some things men want in bed and it is more than just talking dirty. One thing to remember is that men really like to see some enthusiasm. It is nice that they are getting sexual attention, but it is not as fun if their partner is lying there, seemingly waiting for it all to be over. Even if it is a quickie to please your man, show some excitement. They will appreciate it.

Remember to communicate. Tell him what feels good and what does not. Men also enjoy being praised. If they did something particularly well, let them know. There is nothing wrong with a little sexual ego boost.

Finally, remember to take initiative every once in a while. Men like it when their partner initiates sex but still lets them be the man. On occasion, men also like to surrender, which is something we will cover in a little more depth in chapter nine.

PLEASURE TRIGGERS FOR HER

With both women and men, there are parts of the human anatomy that are well-known pleasure areas. However, pleasure does not have to be limited to the parts of the body that are below the belt. Or, when it comes to women, those two that are above the belt. Just like with men, women have several super sensitive spots on their body with higher than usual concentrated nerve endings. Those areas are particularly sensitive to pressure, vibrations and touch. Erogenous zones are huge contributors to sexual arousal and pleasure. Basically, they are the road map to a happy ending.

How many erogenous zones a man or woman have are still up for debate. This chapter is going to cover the seven of the main erogenous zones on a woman. Making it more difficult are that those zones are not the same on every woman and different things turn women on. Regardless of those differences, erogenous zones are pleasurable pressure points that can be explored and used for her pleasure.

The first erogenous zone probably does not need much of an introduction, nor do we need to go into great detail on how to stimulate it. The **clitoris** is the zone with the most sexual arousal and sensitive nerves. Stimulating this zone is the fastest way to get a woman going. There are lots of ways to stimulate the clitoris. Rubbing gently with the pad of your thumb, vibrations, or licking with the flattest part of your tongue are all sure fire ways to make your lady moan. While your lady is on top, you can also press your thumb against her clit and rub in circles with a tempo matching her movements. Just know that simply touching the clitoris is not going to do much. The right amount of pressure or vibrations are what will work best.

The next zone is the **vagina.** In this zone, the walls of the vagina have tons of nerve endings. The inside reacts better to deeper penetration while the outside responds more positively to light touch or licking. Try teasing her by rubbing your fingers lightly across the lips of her sweet spot. You can also blow gently on it in between some light licking and sucking.

The **mouth and lips** are erogenous zones for women. Kissing is a great way to stimulate these areas and they are a direct line of energy to a woman's core. There are many ways to stimulate this part of the body. Taking the lower lip into your mouth and sucking gently, a little nip on that bottom lip is also a great move. Deep, passionate and even aggressive kisses are wonderful as well.

As it is with men, the **neck** is an erogenous zone for women. The nape of the neck is a great place to place soft kisses, give a little blow or flick of the tongue. Just under the jawline and underneath the earlobe are also really great places to land a few of those kisses. Go slow and tease her a bit.

Another couple of body parts that need no introduction and are probably obvious erogenous zones are the **breasts and nipples.** Like most erogenous zones on a woman's body, they are not one size fits all nor is there one particular place that will always be a turn on for women. The breasts are in front, but you do not have to be facing your partner to fondle them. Try something different. Stand behind her and with your front pressed against her back, massage them gently letting your fingers gently caress her taut peaks. From this angle, you have free roam over the entire front of her body. Along the lines of hitting that sweet spot on the breast, when it comes to putting them in your mouth, you also need to exercise caution. The nipples are incredibly sensitive. Some women are able to handle a little more pressure than others. Make sure you know what she likes and does not like before thinking about a little nibble. There are few things that will ruin the mood quicker than pain.

The sixth zone on a woman are the **ears.** There are several nerve endings in the ears from the lobe to the cartilage. They are close to the neck making it easy to go back and forth between the two erogenous zones to really get her excited. The lobes are not quite as sensitive as the nipples, so a little nibble is not going to kill the mood. As a matter of fact, statistics show many women do enjoy having their lobes nibbled on. That combined with the breath being lightly breathed on their neck and ears only heightens the sensuality of this type of foreplay.

The last zone (not in terms of overall number but the last for this book) is the area behind the **knees.** It might sound a bit accessible, but there are several positions during sex and *before* sex that make that ultra sensitive area easy to get to. Before sex, have your woman lie on her back and give her a massage. While you work her thighs and calves, lightly rub that area behind her knees. Kiss them, lick them…any kind of light touch will be sure to drive your woman wild. Keep in mind that some women are ticklish, which is where the right amount of pressure comes in. Ensuring you do not go too lightly will keep her from giggling.

As previously stated, there are lots of erogenous zones on a woman. Those discussed here are the most common and are a great place for you to start. The more time you spend trying to please your woman, the more zones you might discover.

FOREPLAY FOR HER

Let's face it. Foreplay is *not* just about breasts, kissing and intercourse all within about ten minutes. In order to experience as well as share amazing sex with your significant other, foreplay needs to be an integral part of your sex life. We all know there are going to be instances in which time does not allow for foreplay. That is okay so long as it is not on a regular basis. As covered in the previous chapter, quickies will get boring and your sex life will become stagnant. There is an art to foreplay and it comes down to it being a way to woo and court your woman and her sensual zones as well as her arousal.

We will get to some foreplay tips for your woman here in a moment. First, we are going to talk about some of the most important basics when it comes to foreplay. There are three things you should keep in mind.

1. Foreplay is *preparing* to have sex. It is the buildup both parties need and will truly enjoy if done properly.

2. Foreplay should *never* be rushed. The occasional quickie aside, when it comes to pre-game warmups, make sure you spend a reasonable amount of time building up that sexual tension between the two of you. Plan on that being at least twenty to thirty minutes.

3. Foreplay is all about anticipation and sexual arousal. It is about getting your partner in the mood and focusing on pleasure for the both of you. What she enjoys, you need to enjoy *doing* to her for it to work.

Honestly, women can be tough to please sexually. It is not in their genetic makeup to find quick release. Women need a little more time and attention when it comes to sex and foreplay. That being said, there are some things you can do without having to be in the bedroom. It sounds much naughtier than it is. Do not worry. People most likely are not going to know what is going on, which makes it kind of like a dirty little secret between you and your woman.

If you are in public, give her a kiss on the cheek. Nothing makes a woman feel sexier than knowing her partner is proud to have her as his partner and is glad to make it known to everyone around them. Insider tip: that is a great way to boost her confidence and self-esteem as well as a fantastic pre-foreplay trick. Moving on. Another low-key public display of affection (also known as PDA) is holding her hand, putting your arm around her. If no one is looking, give her butt a squeeze. Those kinds of things get your lady thinking about other kinds of touching.

There are verbal queues you can give your lady that will help as well. We are not talking about *talking dirty*, at least not yet. Later on, we will provide some tips on using words to arouse your woman's senses. For now, we are talking about the low-key things you can do either in your house or in public that are not so over the top, onlookers will shake their head in horror. Tell your lady you love her. Compliment her outfit, or how her jeans hug her curves. Tell her that she is beautiful. There is one thing to point out when speaking about the things you say to your woman. Never overdo it and never sound insincere. There is such thing as too much of a good thing. While women do like to be complimented and hear that their partner thinks that they are beautiful, saying it too much makes it sound insincere. Most women do not believe that their pajamas "hug their curves" just right. Know when to use these phrases and use them sparingly.

While you can hit those previously discussed pleasure triggers as part of your foreplay, there are some other things you can do that a woman will really love. As with men, women do love it when their partner talks dirty to them. You will want to speak with confidence when using dirty talk or it will come off as forced and unrealistic.

As we have previously discussed, foreplay can (and should) start long before you make it to the bedroom. Talking dirty is a great way to start. Whether text or in person, take the opportunity to say something sexy to her. Get her turned on and thinking about all the delicious things the two of you are going to do once you make it to the bedroom. Tell her exactly what you want to do to her. Speak low, keep eye contact and go into great detail.

When you get into the bedroom, take things slow. There is no need to get into a rush. It will build that sexual tension that will eventually lead to mind blowing sex. All you have to do is be patient. Start out by massaging her neck and get her to relax. Make your way down over her shoulders and arms, placing an occasional kiss on her bared skin.

Remove her bra slowly as well. The clasps can be tricky, but there is a method that works quite well. Slip your index and middle finger up underneath the clasp. Use your thumb to pinch against the forefinger until you have unhooked the clasp. Most bras have two to four, so repeat depending on how many of those pesky hooks you need to get out of the way. Once the bra is removed, kiss and lick her nipples. If hair pulling is something she is into, you can do that while you give her breasts the attention they deserve.

Save the pants, skirt and panties for last. Going for those first might lead your woman to believe you want to get straight to it. Once the pants or skirt are out of the way, try pulling her panties down to her mid thigh using only your teeth. From there, you can pull them down with your hands. Just remember to take it slow.

Another type of foreplay your woman will love is a sensual massage. When you have removed all of her clothes (bra and panties included), rub her body all over, kissing her simultaneously. When you are massaging her neck and shoulders, kiss her neck and nip gently on her ears. While doing that, breathe heavily onto her skin. It will give her the most delightful chills and make her anxious for you to take her.

The next type of foreplay we will talk about is oral. If you have used the ideas above, she will be ready, but you are going to tease her just a while longer. By this point, you should be at least fifteen minutes into foreplay and now you have a few more to go, but this is the best part.

After the massage, have your woman roll onto her back. Get between her legs and start by kissing the inner thighs. Spend time on both legs, licking and kissing each of her inner thighs. As you make your way up, avoid licking or kissing her sweet spot just yet. Once you have covered both thighs with kisses, move to the inner lips (scientifically known as the labia minora). Gently lick and kiss the inner lips, spreading them slowly then lick a slow line from the base to the clitoris.

By this time, you should have her practically begging for you to enter her. There is one last thing you need to do before you get there though. Use your fingers to tease her a little more. As you lick the clitoris, glide your index finger into her, pulling and pushing it in time with your tongue.

There is a chance she will have an orgasm while you are in the foreplay stage, which is great! If she happens to climax while you are still licking her, blow gently on the clitoris. It is sensitive from all you have done and it will really make her climax that much better.

Now that we have talked about foreplay, we will give wrap up this chapter with a few post foreplay tips and tricks to really ramp up your sex. Once the two of you have gotten past foreplay, there are a couple other tricks you can use to prolong sex and make for an even more explosive orgasm. Starting and stopping is a great way to do this. When you feel yourself nearing climax, have her stop. Let the sexual tension diminish a little and then start again. Do not stop completely. While the two of you have paused sex, continue to kiss her and touch her. That way, you are keeping her senses aroused.

Keep in mind that while men are very visual creatures, women are quite brainy. What we mean by that is, women like their minds stimulated just as much as their bodies. Talk to her, tell her she is beautiful and follow those words up by showing her just how much you think so.

SPICING IT UP! SEXUAL POSITIONS FOR HER

Athletes always say that form is imperative when it comes to performance. Mixing up techniques might help to shave a few seconds off lap time in the pool or it can help score some extra points in the big game. The concept is the same when it comes to sex. The right position usually means the difference between reaching climax and ending up with the female version of blue balls. In this chapter, we will cover positions geared toward pleasing your woman.

The first position is referred to as the *G-Whiz*. Your woman will lie on her back and raise her legs up over your shoulders. (depending on flexibility, you might have to let them rest on your forearms) This position tightens the vaginal walls making it easier for you to hit that elusive G spot. The thighs should be far enough apart that either she or you has access to the clit. Rubbing that is not a necessary part of this position. It is only an option that can be used.

Surprisingly enough, *doggie style* is just as pleasurable for a woman as it is a man. In this position, the woman can determine the depth in which her man can go by adjusting her thighs accordingly. The further they are spread out, the deeper he will go. A tip here is to have your woman close her knees. It will do the same as the G-Whiz position in that it tightens the vaginal walls. Either you or your woman can reach down and massage the clit for added pleasure that is sure to take your woman to O town in no time.

We discussed *reverse cowgirl* previously, but it is great for pleasing your lady. In this position, she is in complete control. It also helps to delay the man's climax, which makes for longer lasting sex. Just like with doggie style, either of you can massage the clit or the breasts and nipples, which will add to the stimulating sensation of her being in control.

Next up is the *corkscrew*. Your woman will lie on the edge of the bed or a bench with her back to you. She will need to lie on one side, resting on the hip and forearm of that side, pressing her thighs together. He will stand and straddle, entering her from behind. If she keeps her thighs pressed together, it makes for a tighter hold on him while he thrusts and it clenches the inner vaginal muscles, making the entry tighter. While in this position, the man can do most of the work, if she presses back against him so that the pace is matched, it makes for an even more mind blowing experience.

Magic Mountain is something you may or may not have heard of. To achieve this, you will sit on the bed facing your woman, your feet flat on the bed with your knees bent. Lean back slightly on both palms to support yourself. Your woman will place her legs over yours with her feet close to your hands. Her position is going to mirror yours almost exactly. In this position, there is not much either of you can do with your hands, but the rocking against your hips with her legs spread will bring her unbelievable pleasure.

Another lesser known position is called the *X-Factor.* The couple will start out in the missionary position. While you are still seated inside your woman, rotate to the right so that your bodies look like an X. You will be just off to the side. That sensation alone is enough to bring her to climax. While in the X position, you are still able to thrust inside her from an entirely new and incredibly hot angle.

These are just a few positions you can use to blow your woman's mind while the two of you have sex. Experiment and find what works best for you. The positions in this chapter are sure to have your woman smiling for days.

ROLE PLAY

Like foreplay and pleasure triggers, role play can please both you and your partner. When we are talking about pleasure and having better sex, orgasms or even strengthening a relationship, being comfortable enough with your partner to explore new avenues is a great way to do all of the above. When we talk about role play, we are not referring to those cheesy scenes in porn flicks. Yes, some of the ideas we discuss might have been used, but there will be no poor dialogue ending in some raunchy sex. Unless you like it that way, in which case I say…go for it. This is about what you and your partner enjoy. This chapter is going to provide you with ideas to get role play started and trust me when I say it is going to be fun.

There are many people who want to try role-playing but wind up tossing the idea because they are not able to come up with the kind of fantasy they want to try. If this is something you have never done before, it is best to start out nice and slow. Simplicity is best. Choose a scenario that perhaps you are already familiar with. Below, we will provide you with some role play ideas to think about. Take a look at the list and try to imagine you and your partner getting into some of these scenarios.

1. Personal trainer and trainee.

2. Athlete and coach.

3. Patient and doctor.

4. Photographer and model.

5. Repairman and homeowner.

6. Student and professor.

7. Client and massage therapist.

8. Potential buyer and real estate agent.

These are just some ideas that will get your thoughts wandering. If you would like, think about what fantasies you had while you were younger. It could be someone in a position of power or authority you had a crush on. Or it could be something like the cheerleader and quarterback situation. The scenarios are endless. All you have to do is think about what you like best and go from there.

People who are new to this concept might be intimidated by the acting part. If that is the case, fear not. There does not need to be Hollywood A list acting complexity when it comes to role play in the bedroom. There is no need for some deep backstory. You can be strangers who have never met before making it easy for you to simply be yourselves. You can also try playing around with power dynamics. Perhaps one of you is the boss and is in complete control while the other is required to submit and follow all instructions.

Now that you have all your fears and worries set aside *and* you have come up with a few scenarios, talk about them with your partner. If you are the shy type and are worried about how to bring it up, do not fear...we have you covered here too. Below are a couple of ideas to start the discussion.

1. Probably one of the easiest ways to open up dialogue for the role play fantasy is to say you had a dream about whatever scenario you decided you wanted to try. Talk to your partner about the dream and let them know how much it turned you on. Chances are, they are going to suggest the two of you give it a try.

2. Look for queues or situations in which you can bring it up. Perhaps if the two of you went to a sporting event, you can mention to your partner that you have always had a cheerleader/quarterback fantasy. You could also use the coach/athlete here too.

3. If having a face to face conversation is too difficult, you can always write your ideas down and have your partner read it later. With technology, you can also send a text message or even an email message. There is a level of excitement sending that type of message.

If you are to a point in your relationship where you are considering trying something new, you really do not have anything to worry about. It is entirely natural to want to keep things exciting in the bedroom. Once you have talked to your partner about your fantasies, ask them what *theirs* are. No matter what their ideas are, make sure you show them the same dignity and respect you wanted from them when you conveyed your ideas to them. After the two of you have talked about your fantasies, it will be time to start planning.

This is not the type of thing that happens spontaneously. In theory, it could, but it would probably be awkward and resemble the cheesy porn we talked about at the start of this chapter. What is awesome about role play is that you and your partner can make it as simple or complex as you want it to be. Role play can be done with words alone, props or costumes. In the beginning, avoid the use of too many props, especially if they are the type you need to purchase for your fantasy. You do not want to spend a ton of money on something only to realize it was not what you thought it would be. (I'm talking about the scenario, not role play. I am sure this is something you and your partner are going to enjoy once you find what works best for you).

In the planning phase, try to share as many details as possible. What parts do you want to play, what actions will the two of you take, where will you role play and when? If it is the fantasy of just one of you, it is okay to tell your partner what you want done, but in order for this to be fun for the both of you, both partners should contribute some ideas. For instance, if the fantasy is the two of you are complete strangers, he could have an idea of how he wants you to approach him or introduce yourself while you can suggest where the two of you will meet. And yes, we are talking about meeting in public. Remember in the previous chapters we talked about those little PDAs being good for foreplay? The excitement of meeting in public to start your fantasy is only going to build some serious sexual tension.

When it comes to planning, we should mention that it does not have to be excessively detailed. Maybe try choosing one of the scenarios we talked about above. For instance, most people are familiar with how a doctor appointment goes. For that kind of fantasy, there does not need to be a detailed script or real planning. It might even be fun to ad-lib instead of planning it in its entirety.

Next, you and your partner are going to want to set your limits. With anything new you try in the bedroom, limits are probably one of the most important things to discuss beforehand. The two of you need to discuss sexual boundaries. For example, if you do not want to be called demeaning names or if anal is off limits, those are the things that need to be discussed before you start your fantasy. During the discussion of limits, you can talk about whether or not a safe word will be necessary. If so, the two of you will need to agree that all action will cease immediately once that word is spoken. Just make sure it is a word that would not be used during the course of your role play activities.

During the planning process, just make sure you have fun. This can build excitement, yet it is important not to take it too seriously. That would take the fun out of it. Getting into the details of your fantasies can be just as sexy as role playing itself!

Finally, we will talk about playing your role. It is time to act out your fantasy and probably the best part of role play is anticipation. You might want to consider drawing things out a while to tease each other. Be oblivious to your professor's advances or stand a little too close to the repairman as he fixes the kitchen sink.

Know that it is entirely natural to be worried that you will be awkward or that you will be afraid of exactly what to say or do, especially in the beginning. Just keep in mind that this is all a fun, super sexy game the two of you are playing. There is no one there to judge your ability to act, so there is absolutely no reason to put too much pressure on you or your partner. If you say or do something silly, laugh it off and keep going. It is always easier to acknowledge something awkward than to pretend it did not happen at all.

Once you and your partner have role-played, talk about how it went. What did you like? Was it a fantasy you would want to explore again or are the two of you going to try something entirely different? Make sure to discuss anything you think did not go as well as you would have liked either. It might be something your partner enjoyed but you did not. If they are unaware that it was something you did not like, they might try to do it in the future. Remember, in any relationship open communication is important. When it comes to sex, voicing your likes and dislikes in *any* situation is even more important.

PLEASURING YOUR PARTNER WITHOUT INTERCOURSE

That may sound like it might not be fun, but there are so many ways to please your partner without actually having sex. Perhaps you are somewhere that getting naked would be frowned upon so the two of you rub up against each other instead. The point of this chapter is to show ways you can achieve orgasm without any kind of penetration. It is a great way to build a deeper bond between you and your partner and it gives you fantastic new ideas to be intimate.

Sex is something that we are talking about much more openly than ever before. The downside is that sex is portrayed relatively unrealistically, especially in film. Porn included. There does not have to be penetration to achieve orgasm. It is a myth that has been perpetuated over the years and because it is something we believe, we take it as truth and do not tend to try new and exciting ways of having an orgasm. A study done way back in 2009 showed that a whopping *seventy-five* percent of women were unable to have an orgasm through traditional sex. A more recent study done by *Cosmopolitan* in 2015 showed even more dismal numbers. Only about fifteen percent of women climaxed through traditional vaginal sex without some form of clitoral stimulation.

In this book, we have talked about pleasure triggers, foreplay, sexual positions and role play. These chapters are all geared toward pleasuring your partner and while the statistics listed above may seem dismal, know that this book is designed to help find new and exciting ways to pleasure your partner. With all of that out of the way, let us get to the good stuff!

Masturbating in front of each other may sound like it would be awkward. However, if you are truly comfortable with your partner, there should be nothing the two of you cannot do in front of or with each other. This is not only something new and exciting, it is a way for the both of you to become more sexually confident with yourselves and with one another. It is an adult form of show and tell that can help you take control of your climaxes in a naughty fashion. There are a couple of ways you can do this. The two of you can discuss it prior to the show. Or, if one of you is feeling particularly gutsy, you can be *accidentally* caught pleasuring yourself on the couch or in the bedroom right around the time your partner is supposed to be getting home from work. Either way, being able to watch your partner pleasure themselves while you do the same, you are going to have a fantastically sexy time.

The use of sex toys is another way you and your partner can pleasure each other without penetration. A simple Google search will yield thousands of results for toys. There are kits specifically geared toward couples. Likewise, there are individual items that can be purchased for him or for her. From vibrators to bondage, oils and imitation vaginas, there are plenty of things for the two of you to try. What is great about toys is if the two of you have progressed to the point you can masturbate in front of each other, you can use some of your news toys while your partner watches. Alternatively, the toys can be used by you on your partner and once they have reached climax, it is their turn to pleasure you. Because there are literally *thousands* of toys to try, you will undoubtedly find something that both you and your partner love. You might even find several things the two of you enjoy.

The next item we are going to discuss is direct stimulation. This is geared more toward pleasuring a woman as it applies to pressure or stimulation applied to the clitoris. This can be done via oral sex, which of course can be done on a man as well. However, direct stimulation does not necessarily mean nothing but oral. There are a lot of women who are self-conscious about their lady bits making it hard for them to climax with oral sex. Instead, try rubbing the clit in slow circles with the pad of your thumb while looking your lady in her eyes. The use of specific clitoris stimulating toys also works well. There is a lot of fun to be had in exploring your woman's vagina. The labia and the vulva have a lot of pleasure sensors. Find what she likes and stimulate her without penetration.

Frottage is another way to achieve climax without penetration. It may sound like the name of a fabulous dessert when in reality, it is something the majority of us did when we were teenagers. Frottage is a beautiful way to say *dry humping.* This is where you rub and grind against your partner either partially or fully dressed. Realistically, complete nudity is okay too, as long as there are no accidental entries. This is an exciting and even unexpected thing to try well past the age of twenty-one. As long as the clothes are on, one does not need to concern themselves with birth control. It is also a great new (and rare) opportunity for the two of you to achieve simultaneous climax.

We are going to cover one more topic before we get a little deeper into partner pleasing sex in the next chapter. The last thing we will discuss here is that of breast orgasms. There is so much attention paid on how breasts look that so many people forget that they are not only lovely to look at, but are sensitive enough for a woman to climax without actual penetration. And, if we want to really get dirty, a man can also have an orgasm by sliding between his woman's breasts. That being said, breasts can swell an additional twenty-five percent when women are aroused. Some are even capable of changing color. When the nipples are licked or massaged, even tapped with a soothing rhythm, it can directly affect the clitoris and vagina making the woman have an orgasm simply by fondling her breasts.

These are just some ways you and your partner can try pleasuring one another without actually having intercourse. Sex is fun, there is no doubt about it. Trying new things can be incredibly exciting and anything that might be considered taboo or outside the box makes the sexual experience (with or without penetration), that much more exciting.

TABOO SEX

Even though sex is a little more in our faces and some things are more socially acceptable, there are things that happen behind closed doors that are considered a little more taboo. Really, that can ensconce anything outside of traditional sex. This chapter is going to talk about three different topics. We will cover BDSM (not the *Fifty Shades* type), voyeurism and tantric sex. These are all outside the box ways to please your partner. Just remember not to do any of them without discussing it first. Especially when it comes to bondage and voyeurism.

First things first. What is BDSM? It stands for Bondage and Discipline/Dominance and Submission and Sado-Masochism. In its most basic form, it is about sexual acts of eroticism as it pertains to domination and relinquishing control. BDSM has gotten a bad reputation over the past few years. The basic principles are meant to be liberating and if engaged in properly, it can lead to mind-blowing sex between you and your partner. What is great about BDSM is either the man or the woman can be in the dominant role or the submissive role. If a woman takes control, it can actually give her sexual confidence a great boost. When it comes to BDSM, it is important to have an open mind, know what your boundaries are (as well as those of your partner), you are going to have a great time with this form of sex.

So, how do you get things started? Talking to your partner about your desire to try BDSM might be worrisome. Really, there is nothing to worry about. There are a few ways to approach this with your partner. First and foremost, it is ill-advised to spring BDSM on your partner. There is nothing more likely to turn them off to this forever. It is best to sit down and have a heart to heart with your partner about your wanting to try this.

If you are nervous about having that kind of chat with your partner, try arranging yourself in a manner that reflects your desire. Bring some handcuffs, a blindfold or some ties into the room. Once again, never tie your partner down without their permission. What we mean here is to say bring them in for your partner to tie you up. If this gives you the green light, take it a step further. Perhaps ask something along the lines of "so, does it turn you on when I hold my hand over your mouth?"

Now that the waters have been tested, and you have been given the green light, you can try taking it to the next level. Next we are going to give you tips on playing the dominator in the bedroom.

No matter who is playing the dominating role, there has to be a clear establishment of who exactly is in charge. You can begin by telling your partner that they are not going to climax until after you have. You can then demand that your partner pleasure you with their fingers or their mouth...whatever it is you desire. This is very exciting to your partner and it will probably turn them on to the point they are willing to do anything you demand of them.

BDSM plays to the senses. Men in particular are quite visual so if you take that away from them, it will heighten their other senses. Put your man in front of you and place a blindfold over his eyes as he kneels on the ground. Tease him with your words and your touch while he is blindfolded. It creates an incredible anticipation. This is so unusual for him that he probably will not know what to do with himself. In a good way, that is.

With BDSM, there are many avenues to explore. When it comes to true BDSM, one partner is the dominant while the other is the submissive. There is no flip flopping back and forth. In a lighter sense of play, you are able to try out both roles. If it is a long-term thing the two of you are going to commit to, there are no blurred lines and one will have to take on the dominant role. It truly is an exciting way to spice up sex both in and out of the bedroom.

Next, we are going to talk about how sexy and exciting voyeurism can be. Again, this is something that absolutely must be agreed upon by both partners. Voyeurism can be an incredibly sexy rush, especially if the both of you are super into it.

If you have ever accidentally caught someone undressing and found you liked it, then that is a form of voyeurism. It is an interest or fetish where someone gets sexual pleasure out of watching another person in a sexual act. It could also be something as innocent as undressing. Voyeurism without consent is against the law and there are no fine lines. If this is something you and your partner discuss beforehand, there are ways to be voyeuristic with consent.

Below are seven ways you and your partner can be more voyeuristic in your sex life. If the two of you agree, these are going to be a great way to bring some excitement to your bedroom and beyond.

First, try using mirrors. The next time the two of you have sex (even if it is the kind without intercourse), use a mirror. Set it up sideways next to your bed. Get the mirror close so you can get a real great visual of what the two of you are doing to each other. It will almost feel as though you are being watched by another couple.

Another tip is to role play. We touched on this in chapter seven and it applies in the voyeuristic sense as well. One of you can pretend that you are a stranger. Perhaps ask your partner to undress in another room while you watch through a crack in the door or the window. As long as it is something that excites you and your partner, it will be a lot of fun.

You can also try going to a strip club together. If there is one close to your home, go together and watch a show, perhaps even indulge your partner (or the both of you) in a lap dance by one of the dancers. If there are no such clubs near you, there is always the option of going to a dance club or rave where patrons will undoubtedly be scantily clad. It does not have quite the same effect of a strip club, but it is close.

Trying a webcam is another great way to try voyeurism. There are websites dedicated specifically to this. A simple Google search with your partner will turn up several results. Once you find a site you enjoy, you and your partner can get online together and watch other couples or even singles. There are almost always plenty of couples or singles to choose from, which is also half the fun!

This next tip might sound odd, but hear us out. Going on a vacation to a nudist resort is a fantastic way to meet people who are likeminded just like you. There are couples resorts and cruises geared specifically toward this type of activity.

The sixth tip is to record yourselves. With technological advances, this can be done on a camcorder or even a cell phone or tablet. You can record your partner doing a sexy dance for you. You can even record the two of you pleasuring each other. It is a good video to keep for your own personal porn collection, which is great for sexual stimulation later on.

Finally, depending on your comfort level, you can watch another couple in bed. If the two of you are staying the night at the home of another couple, you can get intimate with your partner while the other couple watches or vice versa.

Voyeurism is a super sexy and highly pleasurable rush, so long as you and your partner have complete control over your urges *and* all parties are in agreement. If you and your partner are in agreement, it is a great way to pleasure one another in an entirely new and exciting way.

The last topic we are going to cover in this chapter is that of tantric sex. In this section, we will explain what tantric sex is and how you can pleasure your partner by using some of the techniques provided in this final section.

So, what is tantric sex? It is an ancient practice created by Hindus over five thousand years ago. It is the expansion and weaving of energy and is a slower form of sex geared toward increasing intimacy. It also creates an incredibly powerful mind and body connection that leads to intense orgasms. Tantric sex is also referred to as *Tantra* and it is something that can be done by any couple who would like to give their sex life a reboot as well as finding more depth and meaning in their sex lives.

Tantric sex is great if you are looking for something new to try in the bedroom, are looking to become more deeply intimate with your partner, want to reconnect with your partner or if you are looking to find a new and exciting way to pleasure your partner.

The key to good tantric sex is to focus on the art of foreplay, building and building that tension until the two of you are ready to reach mutual orgasm. Naturally, this is easier said than done. Delaying the orgasm in tantric sex utilizes several different methods which include meditation, control of your breath and sensual massages.

Here are some things to do when you are ready to give tantric sex a whirl.

1. Turn down the lights and tune out everything else that is going on in the world.

2. Loosen up! Tantric sex is all about the movement of energy through the body. Giving your limbs a vigorous shake will energize and unlock that energy before you even begin.

3. Keep your actions away from the bed. That area actually triggers a button in your brain that tells your body to sleep. In bed, your body will be looking for that quickie

so that it can settle into slumber. Anywhere outside of bed will help you and your partner find that deep connection, which is what tantric sex is truly about.

4. Find a comfortable spot. Lie down on the floor, look into each other's eyes and touch one another. Take your time and explore every part of your partner's body.

5. Experiment! Try touching in different ways. Feathery type touches, gentle stroking or firm massage. The point is to try and heighten your partner's senses slowly and meticulously so that you are building that tension to a peak without taking them all the way. When done correctly, this type of play can prolong sex and even the pleasure the two of you feel by hours.

6. The last tip here is to not give up. If you and your partner do not make it past ten minutes or so the first time you give it a try, keep trying. This type of sex takes some time to get used to. We as westerners are used to having sex in a certain way which means we have a start, a middle and an end. Tantric sex is not exactly like that and practice makes perfect. In this case, it is also a lot of fun to practice.

With practice, you can let go of all your inhibitions and all preconceived notions of what sex is supposed to be. Eventually you will be able to control your body to the point you are able to delay your orgasm and eventually increase the strength of your climax.

There are some basic exercises you can engage in that will help ease you and your partner into the art of tantric sex. They are meant for beginners and are geared toward increasing intimacy between you and your partner.

1. One of the easiest things to try is the heart breath. It helps the two of you tune into each other. You will stand a few inches apart facing one another. Look into your partner's eyes and place your left hand over your partner's heart. Your partner is then going to take his or her hand and place it over yours. For the first two minutes, focus on trying to match each other's breath. Slow inhales followed by slow exhales, all the while holding your partner's gaze.

2. The next tip is to sit face to face. This actually works best if the woman sits on her man's lap. Wrap your arms around one another tightly and press your bodies against each other. (make sure that at least the top half of your body is nude) Skin to skin contact helps to promote deep feelings of intimacy.

3. Finally, the third tip to start your tantric exploration is to remember to breathe and move slowly while having sex. It also helps to try to avoid positions you know bring easy and fast orgasms. During these slow, methodic movements and breaths, work toward a slow build up of pleasure. The slower the better when it comes to tantric sex. The longer you are able to let those sensations and feelings build, the more intense the climax will be once it is reached.

FINAL THOUGHTS, TIPS AND TRICKS

When it comes to sex, there are literally hundreds if not thousands of ways to please your partner. In conclusion, we will leave you with a few tips for each sex for you to keep in mind when pleasing your partner.

With men, remember that they want to feel desired too. Due to standards in society, women are often the objects of desire and men are considered the owners of desire. Sex is something we make happen which means it is something we can make exciting, fresh and new. A good way to make your man feel like he is the most desirable man alive is to just grab him. Yeah, we mean *there*. It is a great way to initiate sex and it makes your man feel wanted and desired. Morning sex is also a great way to start off the day. He will have a spring in his step and will be smiling all the way to work.

Where men want to feel desired and love the idea of their partner pursuing them every once in a while, women often feel the same. It may sound strange because as we stated a moment ago, women are the object of desire. However nice it may be to have an attractive person take notice, it is far more desirable for the partner to take note of how beautiful their woman is. Tell her and show her regularly. Between work, children and household duties, women can sometimes find it difficult to feel sexy. Holding her hand in public, giving her a kiss on the cheek or even just telling her how beautiful she is are great ways of keeping your woman's confidence levels high. It also triggers those thoughts in her mind and will keep her revved up and ready to go.

You can also try to abstain from sex for a period of time. This is a great way to build some serious sexual tension. Holding off for a few days while in the interim touching and teasing each other will make for a truly orgasmic experience when the two of you do have sex. Do not forget the foreplay, though. Even though you have been building that sexual tension for the past couple of days, you still want to include foreplay. A good thing to remember is to include that pre sex game 99.9% of the time. The occasional quickie is obviously the exception to that rule.

Communicate with one another and provide direction. Remember that your partner does not have the same parts you do. They cannot see inside your head and do not really understand your likes and dislikes. If something does not feel good, tell them. Likewise, if something feels *really* good, make sure they know that too. Keep things as positive as you can when giving direction. You do not want it to sound rude or make your partner feel inadequate. That is a mood killer.

Earlier, we talked about role play, but did you know you can play games with your partner while naked? There are so many variations for you to choose from. Naked twister, naked charades, strip poker…the list goes on and on. You can take any game and turn it into sexy time just by removing an article of clothing every now and then. If you choose to play naked charades, try acting out the things you would like to do to your partner. Along the lines of games, you can also try a Simon Says or Do as I do. Each of you can take turns being in charge of the game. Start by touching yourself and have your partner mimic your movements. It is a super fun way to tease and tantalize.

We have discussed the occasional quickie and there is nothing a man likes more than a quick, unexpected session of naked fun. As a woman, you can learn to enjoy the occasional quickie. In the morning, get up a few minutes before him and prepare yourself. Do whatever you usually do when you stimulate yourself, only stop before you have an orgasm. Then, go out and wake your man up for some really hot impromptu sex. He will love it and so will you!

Earlier in this book, we discussed erogenous zones. There are many more than those we covered so take some time and really explore your partner's body. Find the zone that really gets them going but do not stop once you have found a new one. Continue to explore on a regular basis. It is all part of the fun of foreplay and having sex.

Focus on your partner. It is really easy to get distracted by everything we have going on in life from work and bills to children and family. Believe it or not, your partner will be able to tell that you are distracted. Clear your mind of anything and everything *not* related to sex. Have fun. You do not get nearly as many moments to enjoy one another as you should. When the opportunity does arise, you are going to want to take full advantage of it.

Keep things spicy. Find new places to have sex. Obviously you need to be careful of public places as that is against the law. There are probably unchartered territories in your house. You can try the kitchen counter, the table, the bathroom sink. Up against the wall or bedroom door is always fun.

From new places to new positions, it is always fun to explore new horizons. In addition to Tantra, you can look into the art of Kama Sutra. Like Tantra, it has been around for ages and it is an amazing method to try, especially if you and your partner shy away from things like role play, exhibitionism, swinging or threesomes. Tantra and Kama Sutra are ways for you and your partner to explore one another and realize that special, ultra deep connection that makes relationships stronger and healthier. When we are talking about broadening your sexual horizons, it just means to try something you may not think you will like. After all, you never know until you give it a try. Push your sexual limits and have a great time doing it!

CONCLUSION

Finally, thank for making it through to the end of *Sex: A Modern Guide to Pleasing your Partner*. We do hope it was informative and able to provide you with all of the tools you need to achieve your goals whatever they may be.

The next step is to explore all of these new and exciting ideas with your partner. In addition to the things we discussed here today, there are many more exciting sexual opportunities just waiting for you and your partner to discover them. Keep finding fun things to do to please your partner in the bedroom and that will lead to a long lasting and healthy sexual relationship. Always remember that communication is key. If you do not like something, tell your partner. If the both of you are happy and satisfied, the sex will be amazing.

Finally, if you found this book useful in anyway, a review on Amazon is always appreciated! And Take a look at my other book Kama Sutra a detailed guide to sex positions.

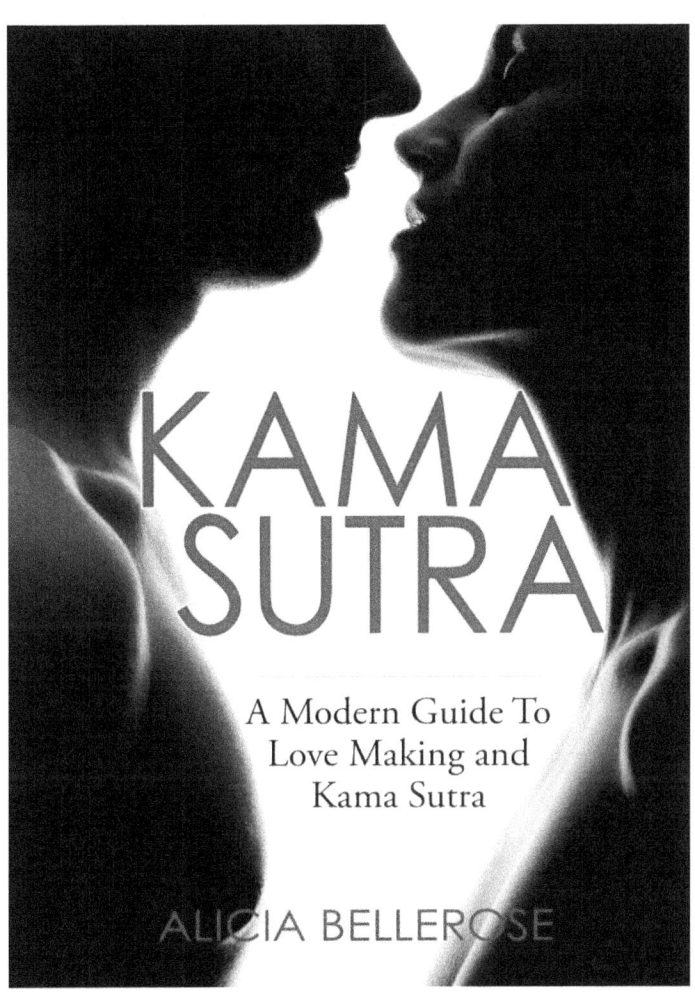

KAMA SUTRA

A Modern Guide To
Love Making and
Kama Sutra

ALICIA BELLEROSE